DEMYSTIFYING PSYCHIATRIC CONDITIONS & TREATMENTS

And Answers To Your Commonly Asked Questions

Vol I

Richa Bhatia, MD

Faculty Member, Harvard Medical School

Table of Contents

AUTHOR'S NOTE

The contents of this book are for informational purposes only. Under no circumstances, should any content of this book be construed as medical or psychiatric advice or recommendations, or as diagnostic or treatment opinion. You are strongly advised to seek the opinion of a licensed physician if you suspect you or a family member/friend is suffering from a psychiatric or a medical condition. If in any medical or psychiatric crisis, please call 911 or go to the nearest emergency room immediately.

The author has no financial conflicts of interest with any products or devices mentioned in this book.

It is worth noting that there are many research findings that are well-known and frequently cited in psychiatry. The author has done her best to reference any findings where the source is known. The author extends her apologies to the originators of any findings, who may have been unintentionally overlooked.

ACKNOWLEDGEMENTS

This book draws on available evidence in the field of psychiatry as well as from my own experience treating individuals suffering from various psychiatric conditions. The available evidence in psychiatry is a product of the work of many physicians, scientists and researchers. In the course of my career so far, I have had the privilege to see a few thousand patients of all age groups, either directly or indirectly by supervising residents and fellows. This book is dedicated to all these individuals and to millions of others suffering from mental health disorders, with the hope that more and more people gain awareness about psychiatric disorders and about available treatments.

This book would not have been possible without the support and encouragement of many people. I owe many thanks to my mentors, colleagues, and trainees who have been a constant source of inspiration, knowledge and encouragement over the years. In addition, I would like to extend my heartfelt thanks to McLean Hospital, Harvard Medical School, Dartmouth College and Dartmouth-Hitchcock Medical Center, Children's National Medical Center and Saint Louis University- each of these institutions has supported me and contributed extensively to my skills and expertise.

Finally, many, many thanks to my family – Nimish, Sushil, Hirdesh, Divya, for their unconditional support and encouragement.

I have changed and invented identifying information and traits in this book to protect the privacy of patients.

INTRODUCTION

There is 'no health without mental health'. Mental health and physical health are closely interconnected. Untreated psychiatric conditions often increase the risk of physical health problems and/or may worsen the course of already existing medical conditions.

Current estimates show that almost 1 in 4 people worldwide may suffer from a psychiatric disorder at some point. Anxiety and depressive disorders are particularly common, with depressive disorders alone affecting more than 300 million people worldwide, according to the World Health Organization. Even less common psychiatric conditions, such as bipolar disorder and schizophrenia, affect more than 80 million people worldwide. This means that hundreds of millions of people around the world are impaired by mental health problems, or are experiencing significant decline in day to day functioning and life-satisfaction because of mental health disorders.

Sadly, millions of affected individuals are suffering silently. Awareness and access to mental health care is limited in most parts of the world.

When an individual suffers from a psychiatric disorder, it is not only the individual who is affected. Often, families and occasionally, even entire communities may be impacted.

I am a dual Board-Certified Child, Adolescent and Adult Psychiatrist. Having seen a few thousand patients of all age groups with various psychiatric conditions over the years, I am writing this book with the aim of dispelling myths about psychiatry and spreading awareness about psychiatric conditions and treatments, with the hope that more and more people suffering from mental health disorders become aware and seek treatment in a timely manner.

Research in the field of psychiatry has grown tremendously over the last few decades, so much so, that most known psychiatric conditions have proven effective treatments. Further research is underway to better understand underlying causes which may guide newer and more effective treatment interventions for these debilitating illnesses.

This book is part 1 of a series that describes common psychiatric conditions, in an easy to understand style, and outlines evidence-based treatment interventions commonly utilized for these psychiatric conditions. In addition, it answers many commonly asked questions that people may have.

With a significant population of the world bearing the burden of common psychiatric disorders, as we move forward into a rapidly evolving future, identifying and treating psychiatric conditions in a timely and evidence-based manner along with preventative efforts to promote positive mental health, will hold the key to a happier and healthier world.

PART I - Answers to Commonly Asked Questions

1. Medications Have Side Effects! Why Would I Want to Take Them?

That's a valid question. Almost everyone taking medications has wondered about this at some point.

Just like medications for other medical conditions such as asthma, hypertension or diabetes, psychotropic medications have potential side effects as well. All medications have potential side effects; that does not mean that everyone who takes a particular medication will experience a side effect. In fact, a significant proportion of people taking a psychotropic medication will not experience any side effects at all.

The decision to take a medication is preceded by careful weighing of benefits and side effects, risks. It depends on your individual clinical condition, its severity, and its impact on your life and functioning.

Untreated psychiatric conditions (such as depression) have been shown to cause harmful structural and functional changes in the brain. If the benefit of taking a medication overweighs the risks/side-effects from that medication, and your psychiatric condition is impairing your functioning significantly, your physician/psychiatrist may recommend a psychotropic medication to you.

You should be forthcoming with your physician about any questions or concerns you may have about medications. Your physician is in the position to help you best if she/he really knows what's going on with you.

2. **I went online and diagnosed myself with ADHD; I want my doctor to prescribe me Ritalin for it. He's not agreeing with me; what should I do?**

It can be dangerous to diagnose yourself! You are not armed with the intricate nuances of medical knowledge to do so. If you suspect you have a psychiatric or medical condition, it is recommended that you bring these concerns up with your doctor. A licensed physician or psychologist can make a psychiatric diagnosis. After a comprehensive evaluation, your doctor will discuss his/her clinical impressions with you.

Psychotropic medications, especially ones like 'ritalin', are serious business. Whether taking a psychotropic medication is going to be safe and recommended for you, can only be determined by your doctor.

Do not pressure your doctor to prescribe you a certain medication. If she/he is saying no to a certain medication, there is usually a clinical rationale behind it. Your doctor went to school for several years to be able to prescribe properly and accurately. Misdiagnosis can mean that you end up taking the wrong medications for a condition you do not have, and in some cases, can be life-threatening if the actual underlying condition is missed and not treated. There have been even reports of sudden deaths of people who misused medications or took them on their own accord.

3. **What is the difference between a psychologist and a psychiatrist? How do I know who to see?**

A psychiatrist is a medical doctor, someone who has graduated from medical school and specialized (completed 4 years of residency training) in the field of psychiatry. A psychiatrist can assess, diagnose, and treat psychiatric conditions using medications, psychotherapy and/or other modalities such as ECT (Electroconvulsive Therapy), TMS (Transcranial Magnetic Stimulation), etc. Psychiatrists may refer their patients to psychologists or therapists for psychotherapy.

A psychologist is someone who has completed a PhD or a PsyD in the field of Psychology, after doing a masters in psychology. A psychologist may specialize in one or various kinds of psychotherapy treatments. In addition, psychologists may perform psychological testing, such as, dementia testing or neuropsychological testing. Barring a few states, psychologists are not licensed to prescribe or manage medications.

Psychiatrists and psychologists often work closely together to coordinate the care of a patient.

In addition, there are licensed mental health professionals such as social workers, mental health counselors, who also provide psychotherapy.

4. I have bipolar disorder; I was feeling great, so, I stopped taking my medications. Is that okay?

You should not start or stop taking prescription medications without consulting your prescribing physician. Many medications have discontinuation or withdrawal effects if you stop taking them abruptly. Not only that, you are at risk for relapse or worsening of your psychiatric condition if you stop your medications abruptly without talking with your doctor.

Bipolar disorder usually requires maintenance medications to prevent relapse of manic, hypomanic or depressive episodes. Many individuals with bipolar disorder make the mistake of stopping their medications when they feel good, only to have another manic or hypomanic episode. Scientific evidence shows that the more number of manic, hypomanic or depressive episodes an individual with bipolar disorder has, the more the likelihood of increased frequency and worsened course of the mood episodes.

5. Do I have to take my medications lifelong?

The answer to that depends on which psychiatric condition you are suffering from, and on the severity of your psychiatric condition.

For example, if you've had several hospitalizations for repeated episodes of severe depression, it is likely that your doctor may recommend taking antidepressant medication long-term.

On the other hand, if you suffer from an anxiety disorder as a result of a recent job loss or other stressor and this is the first time you've suffered from significant anxiety, you may not need medications for more than a year or two if you achieve stability with treatment. The determination of when to stop medications should be made under the consultation and monitoring of your physician or psychiatrist.

Psychotropic medications need to be monitored regularly, and the need to take them or the need for dose adjustment (increase or decrease) needs to be assessed on a regular basis by your prescribing doctor.

6. **My doctor advised me to get ECT treatment. I suffer from severe depression and have tried many medications. Nothing has worked much so far. But, I am afraid about ECT as I've heard so much about it. I saw in a movie that it is really dangerous.**

There is a lot of myth surrounding ECT (Electroconvulsive Therapy). Some of this may be due to how it was portrayed in old movies, such as One Flew Over the Cuckoo's Nest. However, in present times, ECT is performed vastly differently than how it was shown in that movie.

ECT is done under general anesthesia. Similar to any procedure done under general anesthesia, the risks from general anesthesia are there, but, ECT has been proven to be safe and effective for severe, treatment resistant depression and suicidal thoughts, even for pregnant women!

In special circumstances such as if you had a heart attack recently, or a certain kind of brain mass or stroke, you will need specialized assessment by a cardiologist or a neurologist to determine if ECT is safe for you. But, there is really no absolute contraindication for ECT.

Even if you don't have any medical condition, you will be assessed by an anesthesiologist, and undergo tests such as an EKG, lab testing, and in some cases, a brain CT or MRI scan, before you are deemed to be a suitable candidate for ECT.

The good news is that ECT starts working quicker than most antidepressant medications.

7. Will I get dependent on this medication once I start taking it?

There are certain medications which can create dependence.

These are controlled substances (for example, benzodiazepines, certain sleep agents) which have varying degree of potential for dependence. They work on certain receptors in the brain which are linked with dependence. Therefore, use of such medications should be only under the regular monitoring of a doctor. Other commonly used psychotropic medications, such as antidepressants (SSRIs, SNRIs or others), mood stabilizers, and antipsychotics do not cause dependence.

For this reason, FDA has recommended that use of benzodiazepines should be time limited. However, benzodiazepines should not be stopped abruptly as they can cause withdrawal symptoms such as seizures, increase in anxiety or insomnia. Your doctor will advise you on how to gradually taper off your medication if you determine together that it is the right time to do so. If unsure, ask your prescribing doctor.

8. **I plan to get pregnant in the next year or so. I think I should stop my antidepressant now.**

The decision to continue psychotropic medications or not during pregnancy is not a simple one. If you plan to get pregnant in the near future, it is important that you consult your prescribing doctor on a regular basis to collaboratively make a decision about continuing psychotropic medications or not. Your prescribing doctor and you are best familiar with how your psychiatric condition has been. Together with you, your doctor will do a comprehensive evaluation of risks and benefits of continuing a particular medication during pregnancy versus risks of untreated psychiatric condition to you and the baby, to determine further course of action.

It is important to note that different medications pose different levels of risks during pregnancy. Certain medications such as benzodiazepines, or paroxetine pose more risks to the fetus than does fluoxetine. Also, certain times during the gestational period are safer for use of medications than others. In general, it is advisable to exercise caution with use of any psychotropic medication during pregnancy. However, untreated depression, bipolar disorder or schizophrenia can also pose serious risks to mothers as well as babies (including but not limited to, worsening of the mother's psychiatric condition, resulting safety risks to mother and/baby and risk of preterm birth, low birth weight, etc.). All these factors are taken into account while making this decision.

In summary, this is not a decision you should be making by yourself. If change in dosage or switching to a different, safer medication option or discontinuation of a medication is required, your doctor can help you do so.

See the following link from Massachusetts General Hospital, for further information regarding use of psychotropic medications during pregnancy and breastfeeding:

https://womensmentalhealth.org/specialty-clinics/psychiatric-disorders-during-pregnancy/

9. **I was taking Ambien 5 mg nightly, it was working great, but, then, it stopped working. I am thinking of increasing the dose to 15 mg daily. I've not had any side effects from it, so, it can't hurt. Right?**

No, it can hurt. A lot. Again, you must not change doses of medications without consulting your prescribing doctor. Seemingly minor or innocuous- looking dose changes can make a huge difference in your safety and health.

In this example, Zolpidem (brand name Ambien) is accompanied with a black box warning from FDA that the dose of this medication for women be lowered from 10 mg to 5 mg daily, as women have a lower ability to eliminate this medication from their bodies. The FDA warning also highlighted that zolpidem and similar sleep medications can impair alertness and increase risk for adverse sleep related behaviors (sleep walking, sleep driving, etc.) with effects lasting even the next day.

In general, people taking benzodiazepines, other sedative-hypnotics or any sleep agent, must exercise caution with driving or operating heavy machinery the next day, because these medications have the potential to cause persisting drowsiness, impaired alertness even when you think you are awake and functioning fine.

It is also worth exploring and addressing other factors contributing to poor sleep, such as anxiety/depression or another psychiatric condition that may be leading to poor sleep, or by consulting a sleep specialist to see if you suffer from an untreated sleep disorder. Also, sleep hygiene measures, such as having a regular bedtime, soft lights in the evening, no electronic use prior to bedtime, restriction of caffeine and caffeinated drinks, exercising prior to 6 pm, using the bed only for sleep, ensuring comfortable temperature in bedroom, can go a long way in promoting better sleep.

10. My doctor prescribed me sertraline (brand name: Zoloft) for depression. I went to the pharmacy to pick it up and came across St John's wort in the aisle. I think I should take that too, since I've read it can help depression. I know my doctor is not a naturopath, so, I guess I don't need to tell him about it?

Do tell your doctor right away about any herbal or other treatments you might be taking. Even herbal remedies often interact with psychotropic medications that are prescribed to you. Your doctor has the knowledge of interactions that this herbal remedy may cause, when combined with your sertraline, and will advise you about those.

In this particular example, St John's wort is known to be a serotonergic agent. That means, when taken in combination with another serotonergic agent such as sertraline, it can increase the likelihood that you will end up with too much serotonin in your body. This may manifest in the form of milder problems, such as tremors, stomach upset, activation, but, occasionally, can lead to a full-blown serotonin syndrome which can be life-threatening and warrants emergency medical attention.

In addition, St John's wort can cause similar interactions with other antidepressants (older antidepressants such as TCAs- amitriptyline, imipramine, MAO Inhibitors such as selegiline), and even with cough medications and certain migraine medications. In general, St John's wort should not be used with any antidepressant.

11. My boyfriend has ups and downs in mood. I think he has bipolar. Is that correct?

While bipolar disorder presents with significant mood changes, having mood ups and downs by itself does not qualify for bipolar disorder. Mood changes can be due to a depressive disorder, adjustment disorder, post-traumatic stress disorder, intermittent explosive disorder, bipolar disorder, personality disorder or may even represent an underlying medical condition. The mood changes in each of these conditions may be somewhat different and require expert and nuanced assessment by a psychiatrist, psychologist or licensed mental health clinician.

Bipolar disorder is present in 1-2% of the population. Mood changes in bipolar disorder are usually a distinct change from baseline and are episodic. They are accompanied by a decreased need for sleep, with a marked increase in energy during these periods, besides other symptoms such as hypersexuality, impulsivity, and/or pressured speech during these periods. Your friends or family can usually sense that you are not acting like your usual self- this is true even for a hypomanic episode which is less severe as compared to a manic episode.

Therefore, be careful about self-diagnosing. Seek the consultation of a licensed physician or a licensed mental health professional for a diagnostic opinion.

12. I am afraid to mention the word 'suicide' to my sister who is depressed. I am worried about her, but, I think asking about suicide might make her have suicidal thoughts.

This is a myth. Asking questions about suicidal thoughts does not make a non-suicidal person suicidal. Someone who is struggling with depression may already have contemplated or thought about suicide, without you knowing. Maybe, they are afraid to talk about it or mention it for various reasons.

If you are concerned about a family member suffering from depression, support them and urge them to seek the help of a psychiatrist or a therapist.

If you or a family member is feeling suicidal, it is an emergency! Seeking immediate help is of prime importance. Go (or take your family member/friend) to the nearest emergency room or call 911.

The following are some suicide help resources:

National Suicide Prevention Lifeline: **1–800–273–TALK (8255)**, confidential, 24x7. www.suicidepreventionlifeline.org

Crisis Text Line: text START to 741–741

13. My husband likes everything very clean. I think he has OCD.

This is another one of those questions where it is important to remember to not take it upon yourself to become a diagnostician for yourself or your family/friend.

Your husband may have OCD (Obsessive Compulsive Disorder) or another condition, or he may simply be someone who likes cleanliness. The desire for cleanliness, like many other traits, lies on a spectrum. People may be on different ends of the spectrum and still fall within the normal range.

In order to meet criteria for OCD, one has to experience obsessive thoughts or compulsive behaviors for at least 1 hour a day, for 6 months or more, and the symptoms must be significantly impairing daily functioning in one or more life domains. The symptoms should not be explained by another psychiatric, or medical condition.

Your husband might benefit from seeing a licensed physician or mental health provider to review these concerns. If found to have OCD, there are evidence-based treatments, such as SSRI based medications, Exposure and Response Prevention Psychotherapy, which have been found to be effective for OCD.

14. My friend whose husband died a year ago, has been making comments that she wants to die as well. She frequently says she has nothing to look forward to and has withdrawn from most activities. Is this normal after death of a loved one?

Grief is different from clinical depression. A grief reaction involves sad mood, missing the loved one or intense longing for the loved one, but, having suicidal thoughts, frequent feelings of hopelessness or extreme worthlessness are usually signs of a major depressive order rather than a grief reaction. A psychiatrist or a psychologist would be able to help differentiate between normal grief versus a major depressive disorder.

There are grief support groups that can help the grieving person mourn and process the loss of a loved one. On the other hand, if you are concerned about your friend suffering from depression after the death of a loved one, support her, educate her about it and urge her to seek the help of a psychiatrist or a therapist for treatment.

If your friend is feeling suicidal, it is an emergency. Seeking immediate help is of prime importance. Take your friend to the nearest emergency room or call 911.

The following are some suicide help resources:

National Suicide Prevention Lifeline: 1–800–273–TALK (8255), confidential, 24x7. www.suicidepreventionlifeline.org

Crisis Text Line: text START to 741–741

15. My girlfriend is a counselor, so, I don't need a therapist. She can help me.

Having a family member or loved one who is in the mental health field, can be very helpful. This family member or friend can guide you towards the right resources and can help you navigate new and complex systems. However, family members or friends cannot serve as your therapist.

Part of what makes therapy effective is that a therapist is able to be objective and professional. A family member/friend is likely to be emotionally invested in you, have his/her own biases, and for several reasons, would not be the right person to be your therapist.

16. **X medication worked great for depression for my friend. I think I am depressed; I should try it too.**

Different individuals may respond differently to the same medication, so, a medication that worked great for your friend may or may not work as well for you.

It is important to ask your doctor about various medication and other treatment options available for your condition, so that you can make an informed choice. There are various effective treatments available for depression.

In addition, it cannot be overemphasized that do not assume what your diagnosis is, without consulting a licensed physician or specialist. Discuss your concerns with your doctor in detail; she/he should be able to provide you with an accurate diagnosis after doing an assessment.

17. How do I find a therapist or a psychiatrist? I don't know how to go about it.

There are a few ways to find a therapist or a psychiatrist:

- Your primary care physician/family physician/pediatrician may be able to refer you to a therapist or psychiatrist.

- You can find a therapist through this link: https://www.psychologytoday.com/us/therapists

- You can find a psychiatrist through this link: http://finder.psychiatry.org/

- You should be able to find a list of local therapists or psychiatrists covered by your insurance, by calling your insurance company.

18. My child is making comments like 'I don't care whether I live or die'. I don't think he knows much about life or death. He may have just heard someone saying it, right?

Thoughts or comments about death should be taken seriously, regardless of the age of the person making such a comment. Writing goodbye letters, giving away beloved possessions, talking about plans to end life, are additional serious signs of suicidality.

Young children, especially under age 7, may not understand the finality or irreversibility of death, but, may still experience suicidal thoughts. Given higher level of impulsivity among children and teens as compared to adults, they may even be at a higher risk of acting on the suicidal thoughts. There are effective treatments for depression and suicidal thoughts in children and teens. A psychiatric evaluation can be the first step to get your child the necessary treatment.

Call 911 or take your child/teen to the nearest emergency room if she/he is experiencing suicidal thoughts/death wishes/thoughts of hurting self.

19. I tried therapy for a little bit, but, didn't feel like me and my therapist clicked. I don't see any point in going to a therapist anymore.

Sometimes, you may feel like there isn't a rapport between you and your therapist. Therapy is supposed to be a safe space; feel free to share with your therapist what about the therapy sessions is not working with you. Your therapist is not likely to be offended or judge you for that.

Sometimes, what's not working out in therapy may shed light on other underlying themes or patterns in your life, which may be beneficial for you and your therapist to explore and understand together.

Psychotherapy can be transformational and life-changing. Evidence from scientific studies shows that the benefits of good, evidence-based psychotherapy can last for years after the therapy is stopped.

If you still feel like this particular therapist's style is really not working out or not a good fit for you, do not give up. Find another therapist who may be more suitable for you.

Feel free to ask questions, such as what kind of therapy the therapist specializes in, what their area of expertise is, what age group do they commonly see, etcetera, when looking for therapists.

20. My mom is in her 80s. A year ago, she had a heart attack. She doesn't seem interested in anything anymore. She's probably just feeling lonely. Do I do something about it?

Assessment for depression would be important. Depression in elderly people is pretty common. However, depression in elderly is often under-diagnosed or missed, due to lack of awareness, and tendency of the depressed individual and sometimes, the provider to consider it a normal part of aging.

Depression is more likely when there are accompanying medical conditions, such as heart disease, stroke or cancer that are impairing functioning or causing disability.

Depression after a heart attack is common.

The good news is that depression in older adults is treatable, often with psychotherapy, medications or both. SSRIs (Selective serotonin reuptake inhibitors) are often used for depression after myocardial infarction. Certain SSRIs have been tested widely for use after a heart attack, with good benefit. Your mother's doctor would be able to determine which SSRI or antidepressant may be more suitable for her.

Social support and preventing isolation are also important factors in reducing the likelihood of depression after a heart attack.

21. Will my insurance cover me seeing a therapist and a psychiatrist?

Most insurances cover seeing a psychiatrist and a therapist for most psychiatric disorders. You can call your insurance to find out specifically what mental health benefits are covered by your insurance. It is possible that your insurance covers certain therapists and psychiatrists in your area and doesn't cover others. In addition, some therapists and psychiatrists are able to see patients on a sliding scale fee basis.

The American Psychiatric Association and other associations have been advocating for mental health benefits to be covered at the same level as benefits for medical conditions.

22. I tried taking a pill from my friend who has ..... (ADHD/anxiety/other psychiatric condition). It worked great, I want my doctor to prescribe it for me.

It is not only illegal to take a medication prescribed to someone else (at least in the United States), but, can also be life-threatening. Your friend, child, parent, sibling is not you. The same medication can affect your body quite differently than it does someone else's. By doing this, you can expose yourself to potentially serious or life-threatening side effects and risks.

Do not take medication prescribed for someone else.

23. My son likes to eat a lot of sugar. Will this cause ADHD?

A few animal studies have shown increased risk of depression, weakened memory and anxiety with high sugar intake. However, eating too much sugar, while obviously not beneficial for optimal health, is not known to cause ADHD.

The exact causes of ADHD are still being researched. Genetic factors have been implicated in causation, so, having a parent or sibling with ADHD significantly increases risk.

Promoting a healthy and balanced diet for children, in general, is important for better mood, energy and sleep which are all linked with better focusing ability.

If your child is showing signs of inattention, hyperactivity and/or impulsivity on a frequent basis, consult your child's doctor for an assessment.

24. Can I take an antidepressant just when I feel low, and stop it the next day if I am feeling better?

It is recommended that if you have been prescribed an SSRI or an SNRI, you should take it approximately the same time daily. If you do not take it regularly, it is not likely to be effective, as it works by building up in the system over time. Missed doses can lead to discontinuation symptoms, such as flu-like symptoms, stomach upset, nausea, vomiting, headache, sleep problems, mood changes, increase in anxiety as well as a likelihood of relapse of depression.

25. I have tried good doses of different stimulant and non-stimulant medications for my child, since she started showing attention problems 2 years ago, but, nothing has worked so far. What do I do?

If several, different classes of medications for ADHD have not worked, get your child comprehensively re-evaluated by a specialist to revisit the diagnosis, to rule out any other psychiatric condition (attention may be affected in depression, anxiety disorders, OCD, post-traumatic stress disorder, and other conditions) or a medical condition (neurological, vision or auditory difficulties or others) or a learning disorder, all of which are known to cause attention problems. Sometimes, if the above is not helpful, neuropsychological testing can shed more light.

In addition, with the help of your child's psychiatrist, attempt again to gain a deeper understanding of your child's school, social and inner life, to find out any stressors or factors contributing to inattention.

PART II – Psychiatric Conditions and Treatments

Chapter 1. Attention Deficit Hyperactivity Disorder

Example: An elementary school age boy came to my clinic for an evaluation. His parents reported that his school was repeatedly calling them due to concerns that he wasn't able to sit still or focus for any length of time. He appeared cheerful, jovial and smart. As I started talking to his parents, I noticed that he was running around in the hallways, spinning chairs in the waiting room and jumping up and down. When he finally sat down on the couch in my office, it was only for less than a minute. I soon found him in an interesting position with his head dangling upside down from the couch.

I asked the parents and teachers to fill out ADHD rating scales (Vanderbilt, SNAP-IV rating scales can be used). These scales revealed that this charming, intelligent child was suffering from ADHD, combined type. After starting medication for ADHD and titrating the medication to an optimal dose, parents and teachers noticed a dramatic improvement in his school performance and overall daily functioning.

(The above example is fictional, and does not represent any actual person or patient)

Is it normal to have difficulty focusing?

Yes. Every child, teen or adult suffers from some difficulty focusing or sustaining attention at one time or another. Often, when an individual is undergoing major life events or multiple stressors, he/she may experience difficulties focusing or concentrating.

ADHD is diagnosed when difficulty focusing, hyperactivity and/or impulsivity start before age 12, this difficulty is pervasive and significantly impairing school, work, and/or social functioning of an individual, and cannot be explained by another psychiatric or medical condition.

ADHD is both under-diagnosed and over-diagnosed.

The diagnosis of ADHD is often missed, which is unfortunate, given that there are effective treatments for ADHD. On the other hand, there are many people who self-diagnose themselves with ADHD (when they may not actually have ADHD), or assume that they have ADHD, without consulting a specialist or an expert. This can have serious repercussions, as the causes of attention difficulties can be several- ADHD is not the only cause. Assuming the diagnosis as ADHD or something else without a thorough assessment, creates the risk of missing the actual underlying diagnosis.

Diagnosis

There are currently no definitive lab tests to diagnose ADHD. The diagnosis of ADHD is based on clinical suspicion. Since difficulty focusing can be due to various medical and psychiatric conditions, it is important to get a comprehensive physical and psychiatric assessment prior to arriving to this diagnosis, so, that you receive proper treatment for the right diagnosis.

Your physician/psychiatrist/psychologist may ask you to fill out certain forms or rating scales to assess for ADHD. In addition, your doctor may seek further information from school teachers, or may review your school or college progress reports to confirm the diagnosis, and/or to monitor response to treatment.

What looks like ADHD may not be ADHD

Attentional difficulties can be secondary to a wide variety of conditions that are not ADHD. If these conditions are missed or misdiagnosed as ADHD, it can be problematic, as not only does the underlying condition go undiagnosed and untreated, but, you can also be exposed to side effects and risks of treatments that will not address the underlying condition.

Therefore, before concluding that your or your family member's inattention is due to ADHD, it is important to rule out any:

a) Underlying medical condition (such as hypothyroidism, neurological conditions such as, dementia, encephalitis, concussion and others),
b) Anxiety or depressive disorders (which are characterized by concentration difficulties) as well as post-traumatic stress disorder, obsessive compulsive disorder
c) Insomnia or other sleep disorders,
d) Substance use disorders,
e) Learning disorders

The diagnosis of ADHD should thus be made only after a comprehensive evaluation by a licensed physician.

If you were able to focus well prior to the onset of some stressor and developed focusing problems only after a stressor or after the onset of a medical condition or psychiatric condition, the attention problem may be less likely due to ADHD. Treating the underlying medical or psychiatric condition will often resolve the attentional deficit.

See my evidence-based review article at the link below for further information about causes of attentional difficulties:

https://www.mdedge.com/currentpsychiatry/article/114016/adhd/rule-out-these-causes-inattention-diagnosing-adhd

Attentional difficulty is a problem when it is longstanding or pervasive (starting before age 12) and significant enough to be impairing daily activities or academic/work or social functioning.

It is often school teachers, parents or friends who notice attention difficulties first, before the affected individual does.

Types of ADHD

ADHD is of three types:

1) predominantly Inattentive type,
2) predominantly Hyperactive-impulsive type or,
3) Combined type (with features of inattention, hyperactivity, impulsivity.

Who Can Have ADHD?

ADHD can affect anyone. It is more common in boys than girls. Girls are more likely to suffer from the inattentive type of ADHD (i.e., without hyperactivity or impulsivity), therefore, the symptoms may not be as apparent on the surface, and the diagnosis is more likely to be missed.

ADHD has been found to have a genetic correlation. So, if you have a family history of ADHD, you are more likely to suffer from it. On the other hand, having a family history does not mean that you will necessarily have ADHD.

Some studies have shown that cigarette smoking by the mother during pregnancy may be linked to inattention and impulsivity in the child. Similar effects have also been noted with alcohol use during pregnancy.

Sequelae of Untreated ADHD

Untreated ADHD can increase risk of accidents, disrupted relationships and poor work or school performance. Besides that, untreated ADHD can increase risk for anxiety or depressive disorders due to the impairments and debilitation from it.

Treatments for ADHD

Treatment for ADHD usually involves a combination of medications and behavioral or organizational strategies, depending on the age of the affected individual.

Medications for ADHD

ADHD has been found to have strong neurobiological underpinnings, therefore, medication treatment is the first line treatment for this condition. Most individuals suffering from ADHD tend to respond well to one or the other medication class.

Medications for ADHD are commonly divided into two categories: stimulants, non-stimulants.

Stimulant Medications

Stimulant medications are proven to be effective for ADHD. Stimulant medications are either methylphenidate based or amphetamine based. Research shows that both these classes of stimulant medications tend to be equally effective. However, some individuals may respond better to one class than to another. According to some case reports and anecdotal data, amphetamine-based stimulants may have a somewhat higher propensity to cause mood changes or increase anxiety than methylphenidate-based ones.

Stimulant medications are hypothesized to work by correcting the dopamine deficit in the frontal lobe of the brain, the part of the brain that is responsible for impulse control, organization and executive functioning tasks.

Side effects of stimulant medications may include (but, are not limited to):

    a. appetite suppression and related suppression of weight gain,

    b. difficulty falling asleep,

    c. increase in blood pressure and heart rate,

    d. cardiac rhythm changes (your doctor may order an EKG at baseline and at follow-up if you have a family history of early cardiac disease prior to age 40, or sudden death in the family or if you have a pre-existing cardiac condition),

    e. lowering of seizure threshold,

    f. increase in anxiety,

    g. exacerbation or unmasking of tics,

    h. potential for dependence, and

i. potential for precipitation of a manic or a hypomanic episode.

When effective, stimulant medications can confer life-changing benefit for ADHD. However, they should be prescribed after weighing of benefits and risks, and after confirmation of the ADHD diagnosis.

When taken without proper indication, stimulant medications can pose serious risks. There have been reports of sudden death of young adults from misuse/abuse of stimulant medications, so, proper caution needs to be exercised. These medications should be taken only as prescribed, under consultation and regular monitoring by a licensed physician.

My child is not gaining weight at all, although amphetamines are working well for his ADHD. What can I do?

If your child is having a hard time gaining weight while taking stimulant medications, the pediatrician will closely monitor your child's growth using a growth chart and may recommend a nutritional supplement.

Other strategies such as, timing the stimulant medication after breakfast and/or allowing after-dinner snacks (when the stimulant has worn off) may allow your child to catch up on food intake.

However, if your child's growth still remains significantly below the normal percentile range, and assuming it is determined that your child needs medication, your pediatrician may consider alternate medication options for your child, such as non-stimulant medications.

Non-stimulant Medications for ADHD

Clonidine and Guanfacine

Medications belonging to the class known as Alpha-2 agonists, such as clonidine and guanfacine, are often used for ADHD. Both of these are available in long acting (extended release) formulations as well, known by the brand names of Kapvay and Intuniv, respectively. These extended release formulations are FDA approved for ADHD. Studies show that the immediate release versions of clonidine and guanfacine appear to be comparable in efficacy to the extended release ones, once doses are adjusted for equivalence.

How Clonidine and Guanfacine are Different from Stimulants

Clonidine and guanfacine act differently, on different receptors than stimulants.

They benefit hyperactivity and impulsivity symptoms more than inattention.

They are not controlled substances- they do not have risk of dependence and abuse.

They do not possess many of the side effects associated with stimulants, such as appetite suppression, sleep difficulties, increase in anxiety/activation, or tic exacerbation.

On the other hand, clonidine and guanfacine can benefit anxiety symptoms, sleep and tics.

Clonidine and guanfacine, alone or in combination with stimulant medications, may be beneficial in reducing aggression and/or oppositional behavior in children and adolescents with ADHD.

Things to Watch For:

Clonidine and guanfacine require blood pressure monitoring, as they lower blood pressure (as opposed to stimulants which can increase blood pressure).

Side effects may be, lightheadedness, dizziness, low BP, slowed heart rate, sedation/sleepiness/drowsiness. Missed doses of clonidine or guanfacine can be associated with sudden increase in BP, so, caution should be exercised in this regard.

Atomoxetine for ADHD

Atomoxetine (brand name Strattera) is a selective norepinephrine re-uptake inhibitor (also known as SNRI), approved for the treatment of ADHD for children, teens and adults.

Atomoxetine acts primarily on norepinephrine (a neurochemical) in the brain. Norepinephrine is related with anxiety and attention both. Therefore, this medication may be particularly suitable for someone who struggles with both ADHD and some anxiety, or with ADHD alone.

Atomoxetine is a third line medication for ADHD. Atomoxetine may be a suitable option for individuals who may not be able to tolerate the side effects of stimulant medications, or who do not wish to take stimulant medications, or those who have a history of substance abuse, or those who may have had inadequate response from stimulant and/or other non-stimulant medications.

Atomoxetine requires monitoring of liver enzymes, as it has a potential side effect of liver damage. Having a family history of early heart disease or sudden death from heart disease in the family may mean that this medication is not a suitable option for you, or at a minimum, it would necessitate cardiac monitoring. FDA gave a black box warning to atomoxetine (Strattera) that it may increase risk of suicidal thoughts or behaviors, agitation, irritability, and therefore, warrants careful monitoring, especially in the first few months of treatment. (after study showed that 4 children/adolescents per 1,000 had suicidal thoughts and 1 out of 2,200 had a suicide attempt in the atomoxetine group).

Atomoxetine does not cause dependence.

Common side effects may include, but are not limited to, headache, stomach pain, lowering of appetite, nausea, sleepiness, fatigue.

Behavioral Interventions for ADHD

Even though medications are considered first line for most cases of ADHD, behavioral interventions are imperative in combination with medications. Without school-based interventions and a clear behavioral strategy at home, ADHD treatment for children and teens may not be optimal.

For young children age 4-5 years, the American Academy of Pediatrics has recommended behavior therapy as the first line treatment for ADHD.

Behavior therapy usually involves a behavioral plan (based on age appropriate rewards, token economy, structure, consistent/firm limits) and parent behavior modification training.

Feedback:

A high ratio of positive to constructive feedback is very important for your ADHD child/teen. Children and teens with ADHD often receive a high degree of negative feedback at home as well as at school. This can predispose them to developing low self- esteem, getting bullied or even bullying others.

Pick your battles:

Criticizing every annoying behavior that your child/teen engages in, will only serve him/her to tune you out eventually. Instead, in order to be effective, *praise desirable behavior in a specific manner* (saying 'good job' is good, but, not enough- describe the behavior more specifically as well as reward/praise it right away when feasible).

Consequences:

Prolonged time-outs or prolonged withdrawal of privileges tends to feel punitive to a child or teen. Make the consequences and rewards immediate, or as close to the behavior as feasible. A reward that occurs 7 days from the time of the actual desirable behavior will not link the behavior with the reward for your child.

Structure, limits:

Firm, consistent (while empathic) limits and structure can greatly help children and teens with ADHD.

Social skills training, individual or group:

This can assist with social difficulties that children with ADHD may experience. Your child's school may have a social skills group. If not, your physician may be able to refer to such a group in the area.

Other interventions:

Talk therapy itself is usually not considered to be a primary treatment for ADHD, unless it is aimed at helping the child, teen or adult devise organizational strategies or for coping with stressors resulting from ADHD.

Support for parents:

Parents of children or teens with severe ADHD may experience burnout. Support groups can be a valuable resource for parents, in addition to online informational resources such as: https://www.additudemag.com/

School based Accommodations

For children and teens suffering from ADHD, behavioral interventions and accommodations often need to be implemented through coordination with the school counselor or school teacher. These accommodations can be provided via an IEP or a 504 plan (depending on the severity of impairment from ADHD, and/or the presence of any additional diagnoses).

Before devising a special education plan, schools often perform psycho-educational testing, to get a detailed baseline assessment of academic abilities (IQ, working memory, processing speed, etc.) of the child and to rule out any underlying learning disorder, such as reading, mathematics disorder.

Following are some school-based accommodations that have been found to be beneficial for children and teens with ADHD:

a) Giving smaller assignments,
b) Providing more time for schoolwork and homework,
c) Dividing long or complex assignments into sections,
d) Having a timer for work,
e) Providing a school 'buddy' or mentor,
f) Ability to take brief breaks when needed,
g) Developing a discrete signal between the teacher and child to bring your child's attention back (such as a gentle pat on the shoulder or another sign),
h) Assisting with schedules and reminders,
i) Assigning classroom tasks that require movement/activity, such as distributing needed items to peers in class

Most schools are familiar, in general, with accommodations needed for ADHD. Your child's psychotherapist/psychiatrist/pediatrician may be able to talk to the school to coordinate and collaboratively devise more individualized and specific interventions.

When your ADHD Child or Teen Reaches Adulthood

Some teens may potentially grow out of some ADHD symptoms by the time they reach adulthood, particularly the hyperactivity and impulsivity symptoms.

Not everyone who required ADHD medications during childhood or adolescence will require medications (especially the same doses) on reaching adulthood. Some individuals may require medications on an as needed basis, such as prior to exams.

The need for continuing these medications or dosage adjustments should be periodically and regularly assessed by a physician or psychiatrist.

Some resources for ADHD:

http://www.chadd.org/

https://www.aacap.org/AACAP/Families_and_Youth/Resource_Centers/ADHD_Resource_Center/Home.aspx

Chapter 2. Depressive Disorders

What is depression?

Depression is a clinical term. It differs from 'sadness' which is a normal human emotion that everyone experiences at times. Clinical depression, on the other hand, is characterized by pervasive or significant sad or low mood that continues over a certain period of time. In addition, it is accompanied by at least a few other symptoms, such as loss of interest in pleasurable activities, low energy, poor concentration, worthlessness, hopelessness, changes in sleep or appetite, and/or suicidal thoughts.

You don't have to have all of the above symptoms to meet the criteria of a depressive disorder.

What Causes Depression?

The exact causes of depression are still being studied, but, current theories suggest that depression has biological/genetic, psychological and environmental underpinnings.

How Common is Depression?

Depression has a high prevalence, and according to the World Health Organization, 'depression is the leading cause of ill health and disability worldwide' and it is estimated that 'more than 300 million people are now living with depression, an increase of more than 18% between 2005 and 2015'.

Depression is overall more common in females than males, however, it can affect anyone. Males may be less likely to seek help for depression.

Individuals with a family history of depression are more likely to suffer from depression at some point in life, but, having a family history does not mean that one will necessarily suffer from depression.

Depression is Under-Recognized

Depression is often under-recognized, and therefore, under-treated, particularly in certain countries and cultures. Reasons for this may be lack of awareness about the condition, stigma associated with diagnosis and treatment, shortage of mental health providers and resources, and other factors.

According to WHO estimates, less than half of the individuals suffering from depression get treatment for it. This is unfortunate, as millions of people are leading a poorer quality of life as a result of untreated depression. There are effective treatments for depression. WHO has made worldwide treatment of depression a priority.

What depression is not...

Depression is not a personality fault or a weakness. Several scientific studies have proven that depression has neuro-biological (in addition to psychological) underpinnings. There was a myth (and still is, in some places) that if the individual 'just tried harder' to be positive, she/he would not be depressed. Being positive of course is beneficial, however, depression is a condition that requires treatment, just like asthma or hypertension does. A depressed individual may feel like she/he is drowning or weighed down as if wearing lead clothing.

Types of Depressive Disorders

There are different types of depressive disorders, such as Major depressive disorder, Persistent depressive disorder (previously known as dysthymia), Seasonal Affective Disorder, Postpartum depression. In addition, depressive episodes can occur as part of a primary psychotic condition (such as schizoaffective disorder) and are also common in individuals with bipolar disorder.

Major Depressive Disorder

Major depressive disorder is a psychiatric diagnosis. According to DSM-5 (Diagnostic and Statistical Manual of Psychiatry), an individual suffers from major depressive disorder when she/he is experiencing at least 2 weeks of low/ sad mood or loss of interest in pleasurable activities, on most days during this period. Along with that, the individual has at least some of the following symptoms during this time- hopelessness, worthlessness or excessive guilt, sleep changes (insomnia or too much sleep), decreased energy, appetite/weight changes (increased or decreased), concentration difficulties, suicidal thoughts. If these symptoms occur right after a stressor, it may be considered an Adjustment Disorder with depressed mood instead.

An individual may have one episode of major depressive disorder or suffer from recurrent episodes off and on.

In major depressive disorder, symptoms significantly impair functioning in social, work/school or other domains of life. If these symptoms are due to substance use or effect of a medication, or a medical condition, then, it is not called major depressive disorder, but instead, known as substance/medication induced depressive disorder and depression due to another medical condition, respectively.

In addition, there is seasonal affective disorder or a seasonal type of depression, which is characterized by depressive episodes occurring only during winter time and resolving by spring. Bright light exposure treatment in the mornings via a lightbox can be very effective for this type of depression.

Persistent Depressive Disorder

Persistent depressive disorder (previously known as dysthymia) is characterized by depressive symptoms that last for at least 2 years continuously (without more than 2 months of symptom free period during these 2 years). Symptoms may be less severe than in major depressive disorder, nevertheless, they are still impairing one or more domains of life- for example, social life, work or other.

According to DSM-5, symptoms of persistent depressive disorder are low mood for most days during this period, in addition to 2 or more of the following: sleep difficulty (too much or too little), appetite increase or decrease, low energy, low self-worth, difficulty making decisions or poor concentration, and hopelessness.

Again, as part of these criteria, these symptoms should not be secondary to drugs/medications, medical conditions, or another psychiatric condition-if so, they are not considered to be persistent depressive disorder.

This is a treatable condition. At times, an individual may suffer from a major depressive episode in addition to already existing persistent depressive disorder. This is also known as 'double depression'.

Why Treat Depression?

Studies show that major depressive disorder is a risk factor for some serious health conditions, such as coronary artery disease, diabetes, stroke and even some cancers.

Having untreated depression in addition to a medical condition (such as diabetes, heart disease or other) usually means that the course of the medical condition may be worse than usual.

fMRI brain studies of depressed individuals show that untreated depression can cause structural brain changes. Physiological changes in the body occur as well, as a result of depression.

Untreated depression increases the likelihood that depressive episodes may become more severe and pervasive or unremitting over time.

Untreated depression poses the risk of suicide in individuals having suicidal thoughts. Suicide is the second leading cause of death among 15-34 year olds, according to a 2015 report by the Centers for Disease Control and Prevention (CDC).

Treatments for Depression

There are evidence-based effective treatments available for depression, in the form of various types of psychotherapy, antidepressant medications, ECT (electroconvulsive therapy), TMS (transcranial magnetic stimulation) and others.

For mild depression in any age group, psychotherapy may be utilized as a first choice. For moderate to severe depression, usually a combination of psychotherapy and antidepressant medications is recommended.

Psychotherapy

Several studies have shown that effective psychotherapy can change neural wiring or connectivity in the brain, leading to a healthier brain and better psychological functioning. Psychotherapy has been utilized for mental distress and anguish since the 1800s. There are now various kinds of psychotherapy treatments available, and many of them have been found to be effective for depressive disorders.

Psychotherapy may be offered in individual, group, or family format, based on the particular context and needs of the situation.

Here are the commonly used types of psychotherapies for depression treatment:

Psychodynamic Psychotherapy:

The oldest form of psychotherapy is psychoanalysis which is utilized less commonly nowadays. A modified offshoot of psychoanalysis was psychodynamic psychotherapy, which aims to address a condition by exploring, uncovering and understanding underlying unconscious conflicts that may be rooted often in the developmental period. This kind of psychotherapy is effective for personality disorders, depressive, anxiety and some other psychiatric disorders.

Psychodynamic psychotherapy typically runs longer as compared to cognitive behavioral therapy, dialectical behavior therapy or other newer therapies. Psychodynamic psychotherapy is offered by a relatively smaller percentage of psychotherapists and psychiatrists nowadays.

Brief psychodynamic psychotherapy is a type of psychodynamic psychotherapy that is focused on addressing a specific problem and is of shorter duration.

CBT (Cognitive Behavioral Therapy):

Cognitive behavioral therapy or CBT is a commonly used form of psychotherapy that has been studied extensively in the last few decades and found to be effective for depression. It is based on the premise that when an individual is depressed, she/he develops maladaptive thoughts and beliefs which are linked with and perpetuate down mood. With the help of CBT, these distorted beliefs are identified and challenged. CBT typically requires 12-16 sessions. Besides depressive disorders, CBT is also effective for anxiety disorders, eating disorders and other psychiatric conditions.

Interpersonal Therapy:

Interpersonal therapy usually involves 12-16 sessions, and is beneficial for grief or loss, role transitions (related to illness or other life events). The therapist helps facilitate the individual's coping with and understanding of a particular life change/event or stressor.

DBT (Dialectical Behavioral Therapy):

This form of psychotherapy developed as a branch of CBT and is now commonly used. It incorporates mindfulness techniques for distress tolerance and emotional regulation. It can be especially effective for individuals suffering from repeated self-injurious thoughts or behavior. It is also considered an effective form of therapy for individuals suffering from borderline personality disorder.

Antidepressant Medications

Antidepressant medications belong to mainly 3 categories: SSRIs (selective serotonin re-uptake inhibitors), SNRIs (serotonin and norepinephrine re-uptake inhibitors), and Tricyclic Antidepressants (TCAs or older antidepressants).

In addition, another class of medications is MAO Inhibitors which are less commonly used nowadays. MAO Inhibitors, although effective for certain kinds of depression, require stringent monitoring of diet, due to risk of potentially life threatening hypertensive crisis when combined with certain foods. One of the most commonly used MAO Inhibitors is selegiline.

SSRIs and SNRIs are newer than Tricyclic antidepressants, and in general, have a lower side effect profile than TCAs.

There are other antidepressants which do not belong to the above-mentioned categories, such as Mirtazapine (known by brand name, Remeron) which is mainly serotonergic but, works differently than an SSRI; Bupropion (known by brand name, Wellbutrin) which acts on dopamine and norepinephrine, improves energy, lowers appetite, but, may increase anxiety in the short term. Newer antidepressants are worth mentioning, such as vortioxetine (also known by brand name, Trintellix) which acts on serotonin receptors in the brain and is used for depression- it has not been studied in children or adolescents.

Antidepressants carry a black box warning by the FDA of potential increase in suicidal thoughts or behavior, especially in the first few months of treatment, and particularly in children and young people (especially under 24 years of age). No suicides occurred during the studies. However, in the years following this warning, studies showed that the rates of prescription of antidepressants went down while the rates of suicides went up. Later studies showed that the benefits of these medications in treating depression and anxiety disorders overweigh the risk. Antidepressants require regular monitoring by a licensed physician, and more frequent monitoring during dose changes or initial titration.

If you or your family member notices any significant, concerning change in your mood, anxiety level, sleep or behavior when taking an antidepressant, you should call your doctor right away.

SSRIs

SSRIs (Selective Serotonin Re-Uptake Inhibitors) are the most commonly used antidepressants. SSRIs include fluoxetine (also known by brand name, Prozac), sertraline (also known by brand name, Zoloft), escitalopram (also known by brand name, Lexapro), paroxetine (also known by brand name, Paxil), citalopram (also known by brand name, Celexa), fluvoxamine (also known by brand name, Luvox), vilazodone (brand name, Vibryd).

SSRIs work by making the neurochemical serotonin more available in the brain.

Studies show that most SSRIs are comparable in regards to efficacy for depression. However, different individuals may respond differently to the same

SSRI. All SSRIs are FDA approved for depression in adults except for fluvoxamine (which is used more commonly for Obsessive Compulsive Disorder).

How long do SSRIs take to work?

SSRIs take effect over time-they do not start working right away. Most studies show that they take 4-6 weeks to start working, and up to 12 weeks for a full effect. However, some individuals may start experiencing benefits as early as 2-3 weeks from the time of initiation.

Am I going to get dependent on these medications?

No, SSRIs are not known to cause dependence.

What are the Side Effects of SSRIs?

Common side effects are headaches or GI side effects (stomach upset, nausea, vomiting). For most people, these tend to resolve within the first few days of starting medication. Other potential side effects are sleepiness/sedation, potential increase in weight (most studies do not show weight gain of >3-4 lbs a year with SSRIs), increased risk of bleeding (tell your doctor if you have a bleeding disorder or other related condition, and/or if you are due for a surgery), sexual side effects (delayed ejaculation, possible decreased libido), activation/increase in anxiety (especially common with faster dose increase), precipitation of mania or hypomania in predisposed individuals.

Refer to the manufacturer's medication pamphlet for a complete, exhaustive list of possible side effects.

Note: Any medication can cause an allergic reaction or a rash. If you notice a new rash with the start or increase in dose of any medication, consult your doctor immediately. Your doctor may ask you to stop the medication and will make further recommendations based on rash severity. If you notice an allergic reaction, stop the medication immediately.

SNRIs

SNRIs (selective serotonin/norepinephrine re-uptake inhibitors) are medications such as venlafaxine (brand name, Effexor) and duloxetine (brand name, Cymbalta). Desvenlafaxine and **Levomilnacipran** (known by brand name, Fetzima) are other SNRIs. These medications act by making the neurochemical norepinephrine more available in the brain.

Duloxetine at lower doses has more serotonergic than norepinephrine effects. It is best taken with food as it may cause nausea and/or appetite changes. Besides depression, duloxetine is also FDA approved for generalized anxiety disorder, pain in fibromyalgia, and pain in diabetic neuropathy in adults.

Side effects of SNRIs are similar to the side effects of SSRIs (listed under the section 'SSRIs'), but, also include (and are not limited to) a potential increase in BP (especially with venlafaxine). If you suffer from significant hypertension, venlafaxine may not be the most suitable option for you. However, if you and your physician decide that venlafaxine is effective for you despite hypertension, you will require regular BP monitoring and management by your physician.

Tricyclic Antidepressants (TCAs)

These are older antidepressants, used less commonly nowadays due to their relatively heavier side effect profile, as compared to newer antidepressants such as SSRIs or SNRIs. Examples of TCAs are Amitriptyline (also known by brand name, Elavil), Imipramine, Desipramine, Doxepin.

Side effects of TCAs may include, but are not limited to, weight gain, sudden drop in BP when standing from lying or sitting position, constipation, dry mouth, sedation and drowsiness, lightheadedness, urinary retention, cardiac rhythm changes, sexual difficulties such as delayed orgasm, decreased libido.

For a complete list of side effects, please consult the manufacturer's medication pamphlet/guide.

How to Know Which Antidepressant Medication is Best for Me?

The choice of an antidepressant medication will depend on your specific symptoms (for example, someone who is feeling lethargic may benefit from an activating antidepressant such as bupropion; on the other hand, an underweight individual who is not sleeping well may require a sedating, appetite promoting antidepressant such as mirtazapine).

Other factors that influence the choice of antidepressant are your medical history (for example, certain medications are considered safer in individuals with a history of cardiac disease), your family history of response to antidepressants (evidence shows that if your immediate family member benefitted from a certain SSRI, you may have a higher likelihood of responding well to it), and potential interactions with other medications you might be taking.

Your physician can help you find the most suitable option for your condition.

ECT (Electroconvulsive Therapy)

ECT can be life-saving for some psychiatric conditions, such as severe, treatment-resistant depression, suicidal thoughts, or for emaciation due to severe depression. It can also be used for rapid benefit in severe episodes of mania or active psychosis. ECT has been seen to be effective for elderly people with severe depression.

These days, ECT is performed under general anesthesia. The risks from ECT are mostly the same as the risks from general anesthesia. Because it is under general anesthesia, the individual undergoing ECT would not be aware of the electric current that is delivered or the resulting seizure. The seizure lasts less than a minute. Patients are given a muscle relaxant prior to the procedure. ECT is performed by a medical team, including a psychiatrist, an anesthesiologist, a nurse and other medical professionals.

Having performed hundreds of ECT procedures as a psychiatrist, I can say that not everyone experiences side effects from ECT, and even people who do experience side effects, they are usually minor and reversible in the form of headaches, some memory problems (most often short-term), and muscle aches.

ECT is usually delivered in doses of 3 times a week for a course of 8-12 initial treatments. After this course, you and your psychiatrist can determine whether you need a further course in the future, or if you need maintenance ECT treatment for some time. Maintenance ECT treatment is usually less frequent, ranging from once a month to 2 times a week.

TMS (or Transcranial Magnetic Stimulation)

Transcranial magnetic stimulation (or TMS) is a procedure that utilizes magnetic pulses to stimulate nerve cells in parts of the brain to address depression. This process does not require any surgery or general anesthesia, so, patients can drive home after the procedure. TMS is offered in courses of about 4-6 weeks at a time and may be done 5 times a week during a course.

Side effects may be headaches (usually mild), lightheadedness, muscle spasms or twitching. Rare side effects include seizures.

Depression and Medical Conditions

When you are suspecting depression, first, any underlying medical conditions need to be assessed for. Hypothyroidism, pancreatic cancer are some medical conditions that cause depression.

Depression commonly occurs after most cancers, especially those with a high morbidity, due to the toll cancer takes psychologically as well as physically (likely through effect of cytokines and immune dysregulation). Pancreatic cancer is one type of cancer where depression is much more common and can even precede physical manifestations of the disease.

It is now scientifically proven that depression itself can increase risk of not only heart disease, but also, of cancer and dementia.

Treatment of depression in patients with cancer or after a heart attack is important and can be achieved through psychotherapy and/or antidepressant medications. Such treatment can significantly improve quality of life and even likelihood of adherence with treatment of the medical condition.

Do Children Get Depressed?

Yes, children and teens can, and do suffer from depression.

Depression in children manifests more often in the form of irritability or even anger. School problems, especially new or recent onset, may be due to depression. Social withdrawal, decreased interest in fun activities, talking about dying or suicide, rejection hypersensitivity, somatic symptoms such as frequent pains and aches, running away from home or talking about it, changes in energy, sleep or appetite may be signs of depression in this age group.

According to the Centers for Disease Control and Prevention (CDC) report, suicide was the third leading cause of death among individuals age 10-14 in the United States in 2015.

According to current evidence, psychotherapy is the treatment of choice for children and adolescents with mild to moderate depression. Cognitive behavioral therapy (CBT) may be used for children and teens older than age 11. For younger children, behavioral therapy, child directed play therapy, psychodynamic psychotherapy may be the kinds of psychotherapies utilized, depending on the age, psychological mindedness of the child/teen and the nature of the depressive condition. A combination of CBT and SSRI medications, is the treatment of choice for moderate to severe depression in children and adolescents.

A Word About Postpartum Depression

Postpartum depression is more than the 'baby blues' that many mothers experience after the birth of a child. Baby blues are characterized by crying spells, mood swings, and anxiety. On the other hand, women with postpartum depression may experience feelings of hopelessness, excessive guilt or worthlessness, loss of interest in pleasurable activities, thoughts of suicide, or even thoughts of hurting the baby, in addition to other depressive symptoms. Mood changes in postpartum depression tend to be more pervasive and significant than those in baby blues.

Postpartum depression is not uncommon. It is a serious condition, posing risks to both the mother and the infant, if untreated. Therefore, it warrants treatment and timely assessment by a licensed mental health clinician.

Women at higher risk for postpartum depression are those with a prior history of depression, family history of depression, a medically complicated pregnancy or delivery, lack of spousal or social support, and presence of other stressors during pregnancy.

Treatment for postpartum depression can be through psychotherapy and/or medications. Your doctor will advise you on breastfeeding if you take an antidepressant medication during this period. Certain antidepressants have been shown to be secreted in lesser amounts in breast milk as compared to others, and are therefore, considered safer if you plan to breastfeed. Social, family support is obviously a key factor that can help the mother recover optimally.

Other Things You Can Do in Addition, to Combat Depression

Exercise:

Exercise has been shown to be the strongest protective factor for depression, according to research. Moderate, aerobic exercise has the best evidence in decreasing severity of depression.

Act Opposite to Your Negative Emotion:

This is a DBT (Dialectical Behavior Therapy) mantra. For example, if you feel like isolating (or in other words, this is what your negative emotion is telling you), do not isolate. Try to socialize instead. It may feel like a huge burden in the beginning when you try to socialize, but, it is likely to help you feel better, whereas, isolating is likely to worsen depression in the long run.

Sleep Well:

If you want good mental health, sleeping well at night is of utmost importance. Chronically deficient sleep affects brain function and can even be dangerous for your physical and mental health, through increased risk of accidents, memory problems, bipolar disorder exacerbation, worsening of depressive and anxiety symptoms, and other medical risks. Many studies show that regular and adequate sleep significantly helps mood, energy, and concentration.

Chapter 3. Anxiety Disorders

Anxiety disorders are the most common psychiatric disorders. Anxiety is a normal evolutionary reaction to perceived dangers or threat, but, when anxiety becomes excessive, uncontrolled or exaggerated on a frequent basis, then, it starts impairing the functioning of the individual and takes the form of a disorder.

Anxiety disorders can be paralyzing- people suffering from severe anxiety disorders may excessively avoid triggering situations, sometimes for years.

Anxiety disorders can go hand in hand with depressive disorders- it is not uncommon for them to co-exist.

In order to diagnose an anxiety disorder, the first step is an evaluation by a physician to rule out an underlying medical condition. Certain medical conditions, such as hyperthyroidism, pheochromocytoma, cardiac and lung diseases can mimic symptoms of anxiety disorders or cause anxiety.

Types of Anxiety Disorders

The following are some of the types of anxiety disorders:

Generalized Anxiety Disorder

This disorder is characterized by excessive worrying about multiple themes on most days, for at least 6 months.

The individual finds it hard to control the worry or get rid of the worrisome thoughts.

In addition, according to the Diagnostic and Statistical Manual of Psychiatry (DSM-5), at least 3 of the following symptoms are present:

Irritability
Fatigue
Difficulty concentrating
Feeling restless or on edge
Sleep difficulties
Muscle tension

Symptoms that are due to the effects of drugs or medications, or a medical condition (hyperthyroidism is commonly linked with anxiety or panic) or due to another psychiatric disorder, are not considered to be generalized anxiety disorder. Certain medications such as decongestants, some migraine medications (such as ergotamine) can cause or increase anxiety or panic-like symptoms.

Social Anxiety Disorder

An individual is said to suffer from social anxiety disorder or social phobia when there is excessive fear or worry about being judged, embarrassed/humiliated or evaluated in social situations, for at least 6 months. The individual avoids or bears most social situations with great distress, fear or anxiety. These symptoms cause significant distress or impairment in social, occupational or other domains of functioning.

In order to meet criteria for social anxiety disorder, according to the Diagnostic and Statistical Manual of Psychiatry (DSM-5), these symptoms should not be due to drugs/medications, a medical condition or another psychiatric condition.

Social anxiety disorder can be disabling, as the individual tends to avoid most social situations, thereby, perpetuating the fear and avoidance even further. The more one avoids, the more the fear and avoidance burgeons- it is a vicious cycle.

Panic Disorder

Panic disorder is characterized by repeated panic attacks. In addition, according to the Diagnostic and Statistical Manual of Psychiatry (DSM-5), at least one of the panic attacks is followed by a fear of having a panic attack in the future or intense avoidance of the panic trigger, for at least a month.

What is a Panic Attack?

A panic attack is a sudden, abrupt increase in fear or anxiety that peaks within minutes, and involves four or more of the following symptoms, according to the Diagnostic and Statistical Manual of Psychiatry (DSM-5):

Palpitations, racing or pounding heart
Sweating
Shaking/trembling
Nausea or GI distress
Chest pain
Shortness of breath
Feeling dizzy, lightheaded
Sensation of choking
Numbness or tingling
Feelings of being out of touch with reality or out of body sensation
Fear of losing control

Sense of impending doom/fear of dying

Other Anxiety Disorders:

There are other anxiety disorders such as **Agarophobia** (characterized by fear of being in certain spaces such as open or closed spaces, or fear of being outside of home). In agarophobia, there is excessive avoidance of these triggering places to the point that symptoms are debilitating.

Separation Anxiety Disorder is more common in children, but, can also be present in adults. It involves excessive concern, fear or significant distress around separation from attachment figures along with some of the following: frequent nightmares, excessive worry about harm coming to said attachment figure, and refusal to be away from this person to go to school, work or other activities such as sleepovers. Treatment in the case of children involves behavioral interventions with both the child and parent.

Treatments for Anxiety Disorders

Anxiety disorders have effective, evidence-based treatments, including psychotherapy and/or medications.

CBT or Cognitive Behavioral Therapy has the most evidence among psychotherapies, for anxiety disorders. CBT works by challenging negative automatic thoughts and related maladaptive beliefs that are underlying and perpetuating symptoms.

CBT is typically offered in weekly session for about 12-16 weeks.

CBT is effective for generalized anxiety disorder, specific or simple phobia, panic disorder and social anxiety disorder.

Other branches of CBT, such as Rational Emotive Therapy may be beneficial for some types of anxiety symptoms as well.

Psychodynamic psychotherapy has not been researched as much as CBT, but, it is effective for anxiety disorders. Treatment typically lasts longer, usually >6 months. It involves exploration and examination of underlying unconscious conflicts, identification of repeated themes and patterns in the individual's life as well as an understanding of the individual's relationships to primary attachment figures and how these might be contributing to the present symptoms.

Medications for Anxiety Disorders

SSRIs (Selective serotonin re-uptake inhibitors) are the first line medications for the treatment of anxiety disorders. SSRIs and SNRIs are commonly known as 'antidepressants', but, that term is really a misnomer because 'antidepressants' are proven to be effective and widely used for anxiety disorders as well. So, don't be too surprised when your doctor recommends an 'antidepressant' to treat anxiety.

Escitalopram is FDA approved for generalized anxiety disorder, fluoxetine is FDA approved for panic disorder, sertraline is FDA approved for panic disorder and social anxiety disorder. Also, not having FDA approval in case of an SSRI does not necessarily mean that it may not be effective for a particular anxiety disorder. Most SSRIs have been widely tested for various anxiety disorders.

SNRIs (serotonin and norepinephrine reuptake inhibitors) are used for treatment of anxiety disorders as well. Venlafaxine extended release (also known by brand name, Effexor XR) has received FDA approval for treatment of generalized anxiety disorder, so, has duloxetine.

When treating anxiety disorders, your physician or psychiatrist may start an SSRI or SNRI at a lower dose and increase the dose more slowly and to a higher level eventually, as compared to treating a depressive disorder.

Buspirone, which acts on serotonin receptors through a different mechanism, also has some efficacy for moderate generalized anxiety disorder and is FDA approved. It can be used alone or in combination with an SSRI. When combined with an SSRI, it has been shown to boost the antidepressant effect of an SSRI. Buspirone has a relatively low side effect profile and does not cause dependence. It needs to be taken on a daily basis to have effect.

Older antidepressants (Tricyclic Antidepressants or TCAs, eg. amitriptyline) may be beneficial for treatment of anxiety disorders, but, are used less commonly due to their relatively higher side effect profile.

(See chapter on Depressive Disorders for further details about side effects, risks of SSRIs, SNRIs, and TCAs).

Propranolol, which is a medication that was first used as an antihypertensive, has been found effective for social anxiety disorder. Some of the common side effects are low BP, sedation/tiredness, lightheadedness/dizziness, slowed heartbeat, mood changes. It can be used on a daily or as needed basis.

Other medications such as hydroxyzine (an antihistamine), gabapentin (anticonvulsant) may be used off label for treatment of anxiety symptoms.

A Word About Benzodiazepines

Benzodiazepine medications, such as clonazepam, lorazepam, diazepam and alprazolam, are used quite commonly for treatment of anxiety disorders. However, their use is recommended by the FDA for short term only. There may be occasional exceptions to this- ask your doctor if unclear.

The reason that their use has been recommended for short term is that long term use can increase risk of dependence and even lead to memory difficulties. Benzodiazepines work rapidly as compared to SSRIs, but, they are not effective for long-term management of anxiety. Over time, people are likely to need higher doses to achieve the same effect.

In any case, do not stop your benzodiazepine medication abruptly or suddenly. Doing so can cause withdrawal symptoms, including but not limited to, seizures, increased anxiety, insomnia or others.

Benzodiazepines can cause drowsiness, sleepiness, and increase risk of falls. So, caution should be exercised with use of benzodiazepines in elderly who may already be at risk for falls due to fragile health, multiple medications and potential medication interactions. Benzodiazepine medications have not been studied for safety and efficacy in children.

Individuals taking benzodiazepines are advised to not drive or operate heavy machinery after use of these medications, as attention and alertness can be impaired even several hours after taking these. Also, benzodiazepine use should not be combined with alcohol use, due to risk of life threatening respiratory and central nervous system suppression.

The choice of a medication for treatment of anxiety disorders will depend on the specific condition, medical history, presence of any other psychiatric conditions, potential of interactions with other current medications and other factors such as symptom severity.

Chapter 4. Eating Disorders

According to the National Association of Anorexia Nervosa and Associated Disorders, about 30 million people in the United States suffer from an eating disorder. Eating disorders result from a conglomeration of biological, psychological and environmental factors. Often, an individual suffering from an eating disorder has a parent or another family member with an eating disorder.

You may have heard of eating disorders such as anorexia nervosa and bulimia. Individuals suffering from anorexia or bulimia tend to be secretive about these conditions. Therefore, awareness about these conditions can help early recognition and treatment.

Medical Sequelae and Complications of Eating Disorders

Anorexia and bulimia can increase the likelihood of dehydration and other electrolyte anomalies, decreased blood sugar, anemia, low blood pressure, hypothermia, to name a few physiological changes. Purging can lead to an imbalance in the body's potassium level, increasing risk of seizures.

Slowed heart rate, heart rhythm abnormalities are common in anorexia and bulimia. These can place the often malnourished or dehydrated individual at life threatening risks (eg risk of cardiac arrest), therefore, the need for testing and treatment is high.

The hormonal system is affected as well. Often, individuals with anorexia will stop having menstrual periods for months at a time.

Because individuals with eating disorders often hide their symptoms, these conditions may not come to light until they are advanced. Cardiac complications, osteoporosis and other sequelae can occur as a result of severe anorexia nervosa. Osteoporosis can negatively impact bone growth in growing children and teens and is an irreversible complication of anorexia nervosa.

Eating disorders are often accompanied by depressive and/or anxiety disorders. Suicide or suicidal thoughts are not uncommon among people suffering from eating disorders. Treatment with psychotherapy and SSRIs, other psychotropic medications is often needed, to address these comorbid conditions.

With early identification and treatment, complications of eating disorders can be averted.

Types of Eating Disorders

Anorexia Nervosa:

You've probably heard of Anorexia. Anorexia nervosa, when untreated, has the highest mortality rate of all psychiatric conditions. It is more common in females.

Individuals suffering from anorexia display a neurotic degree of perfectionism, rigidity, and a strong need for control which is exercised through food restriction or purging behaviors.

Most females care about their appearance, but, individuals suffering from these disorders are excessively pre-occupied and concerned about their body image. They strongly believe that they are 'fat', when in fact, they may be underweight or even emaciated.

They may go to extreme lengths to be below a certain weight, by exercising excessively, dieting, self-induced vomiting, or even using laxatives or other substances.

There are two types of anorexia nervosa- restricting type, and binging-purging type.

Bulimia:

Bulimia involves binging and purging, however, individuals with bulimia have closer to normal body weight, as compared to individuals with anorexia who are significantly underweight. Strong desire for thinness and body image distortion are present.

Purging is usually via self-induced forceful vomiting or use of laxatives/other medications to lose weight.

Frequent purging can manifest in the form of swelling of parotids (which are a type of salivary glands), changes in intestinal enzyme activity, impact on hormonal and electrolyte balance, and effect on several other organ systems.

Mood swings and depression are common among people suffering from bulimia. Substance use disorders often co-exist along with bulimia.

Bulimia is treatable. If untreated, serious, potentially life-threatening complications can ensue.

Binge Eating disorder:

Binge eating disorder is the most common eating disorder among adults in the United States. According to the National Association of Anorexia Nervosa and Associated Disorders, it is present in about 3% of individuals.

Binge eating disorder is a condition in which individuals consume large, greater than normal portions of food on a recurrent basis, at least once a week for 3 months. This food is consumed rapidly, within a small amount of time, even when not hungry.

Individuals with binge eating disorder experience guilt and shame after episodes of binge eating, and also may experience physical discomfort from binge eating. They do not purge.

Binge eating disorder is often accompanied by anxiety, substance use and/or depressive disorders.

Lab testing for Eating Disorders

Your physician may perform lab tests, such as a complete blood count, thyroid panel, liver function tests, electrolyte levels to assess for and monitor an eating disorder. Your doctor will likely do an EKG to check for any cardiac rhythm disturbances. A bone density scan may be done to assess for osteoporosis, if an affected individual has been severely underweight for a year or more.

Treatments for Eating Disorders

Levels of Treatment: Eating disorders may be treated in outpatient, partial hospital, residential, inpatient psychiatric or inpatient medical levels of care, depending on the severity of the disorder. Treatment emphasizes development of normal eating patterns, and in case of anorexia nervosa, the emphasis is also on weight restoration.

Team approach: Treatment of eating disorders requires a team approach, involving a psychiatrist, a primary care physician/pediatrician, a psychologist, a nutritionist and a cardiologist or other specialist if needed.

What Kind of Therapy is best for Eating Disorders?

A cornerstone of eating disorder treatment is individual CBT (Cognitive Behavioral Therapy), which has been shown by a number of studies, to have substantial benefit in both anorexia and bulimia. CBT is usually offered in weekly sessions for anywhere from 12-40 sessions, depending on how severe or impairing the eating disorder is. Initially, the sessions may be two times a week, to establish rapport and build momentum. In a residential or partial hospital setting, the frequency of psychotherapy is increased to three times a week or even daily in some situations.

CBT works by challenging maladaptive and dysfunctional beliefs around body image, food, self-esteem. There are also a number of studies showing benefit of CBT for depressive and anxiety symptoms, which individuals with eating disorders commonly suffer from.

For children and teens suffering from eating disorders, family psychotherapy is an important piece of channeling the family's resources to help the child or teen to move forward.

In addition, mindfulness-based psychotherapies, self-compassion cultivation can help address maladaptive perfectionistic tendencies.

For children and teens, treatment may also involve an assessment and re-training of parent eating habits and behaviors if maladaptive.

Medications for Eating Disorders:

There is a dearth of FDA approved medications for eating disorders. More controlled studies are needed in this direction.

Medications for Anorexia:

Antidepressants as well as atypical antipsychotics have been used off-label with mixed success for anxiety, depressive symptoms, fixed beliefs and weight gain in anorexia nervosa.

Medications, such as SSRIs (Selective Serotonin Re-Uptake Inhibitors), are often used in combination with CBT, particularly when symptoms are greater than mild to moderate. In severe or refractory cases of anorexia nervosa, atypical antipsychotics may be used (off label) for short-term, to assist with cognitive distortions or fixed beliefs (around eating and body image) that reach delusional proportions. However, studies on use of atypical antipsychotics are small and given the high side effect profile, the use of these medications needs to be monitored regularly.

Medications for Bulimia:

Fluoxetine (Prozac) is FDA approved for bulimia. Other antidepressants (SSRIs and older antidepressants, such as imipramine) have had some studies showing benefit in bulimia. Topiramate has been used off label for both bulimia and binge eating disorder.

Lisdexamfetamine (Vyvanse) is FDA approved for binge eating disorder.

What We Can Do as a Society to Improve Body Image:

An unhealthy notion of desirable body type is commonly projected by popular media. Adolescents, being suggestible and not yet having a stable sense of self, are often influenced by this projection growing up. Millions of teens grow up with an unrealistic image of desirable body type. Although there are genetic, biological and other psychological factors that predispose an individual to developing an eating disorder, creating a healthier body image for growing children and teens throughout the world is a worthwhile goal.

As a society, we can help to curb this by educating and exposing children and teens to a healthier body image, both via media and via appropriate modeling of eating behaviors at home and school.

Encouraging and educating children and adolescents about healthy eating and a healthy lifestyle, without an excessive focus on weight, can go a long way in attaining this.

Chapter 5. Psychotic Disorders

Psychotic disorders are disorders of thought and often of reality testing. These conditions are less common than other psychiatric conditions, but, when present, can be significantly impairing to the life of the affected person and family.

Are Psychotic Symptoms Always Psychiatric?

No. Psychotic symptoms can be due to a primary psychiatric condition, such as, schizophrenia, schizoaffective disorder, bipolar disorder, delusional disorder, or they can be secondary to a medical condition, as in the case of delirium, tumors, masses or even infections in the brain, and other. Therefore, it is important to rule out a medical condition in the case of anyone presenting with new-onset psychotic symptoms.

Addressing and treating the underlying root cause is important when the psychotic symptoms are a manifestation of any underlying medical condition.

Psychotic symptoms can also result from use of illicit substances such as cocaine, methamphetamine and from use/misuse of certain medications such as steroids.

Psychosis is rare in childhood. If psychotic symptoms emerge during childhood, the special importance of a comprehensive medical evaluation cannot be overemphasized. A brain MRI may be done in such a situation, especially if there is no family history of schizophrenia or other psychotic disorders.

If someone you know is experiencing difficulty distinguishing between what's real or not, and seems to be exhibiting bizarre behavior, it is best to get that individual evaluated comprehensively by a psychiatrist.

Treatment for psychotic symptoms can be provided in various settings- such as inpatient, outpatient, residential, ER and other.

In this chapter, we will be discussing various psychotic disorders.

Schizophrenia

Let's talk a bit about schizophrenia. I'm sure you've heard the term often.

How Common Is It?

Schizophrenia is present in ~1% of the population.

Age of Onset:

The common age of onset is between 15 and 25 years for men, and between 20-30 years of age for women.

What are Common Symptoms of Schizophrenia?

Common symptoms of schizophrenia are delusions, paranoia, hallucinations (commonly in the form of 'voices'), disorganized speech, or disorganized behavior. Many patients with schizophrenia suffer from depressive symptoms, social withdrawal, and cognitive difficulties as well. Not all of these symptoms need to be present for a diagnosis of schizophrenia.

Example of Distorted Reality Testing:

An individual suffering from schizophrenia may believe that he/she is living on the planet Venus and be out of touch with reality.

Example of Delusions:

An individual may hold a false, fixed belief that people are organizing to persecute him/her, or that there are insects crawling on the individual's skin, even when no evidence for any of this exists.

Example of Hallucinations:

Hallucinations in schizophrenia are commonly auditory. An individual affected with hallucinations may appear to be talking to people who are not there or may hear voices talking to him/her or to each other, that nobody else can hear.

Correcting Old Myths:

In olden days, it was believed that schizophrenia was caused by a mother being too 'cold' towards her child. Schizophrenia is not due to how a mother behaves towards her child. Research has proven that this is a myth and that schizophrenia is a complex condition with strong biological underpinnings. Its exact causation is still being researched and understood.

Schizophrenia has a higher rate of occurrence if there is a history of schizophrenia in the family.

Treatment for Schizophrenia

Antipsychotic medications are the cornerstone of treatment for schizophrenia. Supportive and other psychotherapy can help manage stressors and depressive, anxiety symptoms related to the illness, however, medications are key, especially if active psychotic symptoms are present. With adequate treatment and community support, many individuals with schizophrenia can have a decent level of functioning.

A Word About Antipsychotic Medications

Antipsychotic medications tend to be very effective and can be life-changing in resolving the psychotic symptoms of schizophrenia. They fall into two broad categories- older or typical antipsychotics and newer or atypical antipsychotics.

How Do Antipsychotic Medications Work?

Dopamine is often hypothesized to be the neurochemical underlying the pathology of psychotic disorders. Antipsychotic medications help to regulate the dopamine level in the brain, thereby, facilitating remission of psychotic symptoms.

Newer antipsychotics, also known as atypical antipsychotics, are aripiprazole, olanzapine, quetiapine, risperidone, ziprasidone, lurasidone and others. Potential side effects are weight gain, abdominal obesity, increase in blood sugar, increase in cholesterol (also known as metabolic syndrome), and therefore, require periodic monitoring of lipid panel.

These medications can also cause abnormal involuntary movements or stiffness of neck, tongue, arms, legs or other body parts however, the likelihood of this side effect is less with atypical antipsychotics than with older antipsychotics such as haloperidol. This side effect goes away if one stops the medication, or by taking diphenhydramine (known by brand name, Benadryl) or benztropine (brand name, Cogentin). If one takes an antipsychotic medication for several years, there is a risk of involuntary movements of the tongue and mouth, known as tardive dyskinesia. Several antipsychotics can cause sleepiness, lightheadedness, and some sexual side effects.

Risperidone can cause an increase in the level of a hormone called prolactin, which can result in breast growth in males. This hormone's level needs to be checked on a periodic basis if taking risperidone. There is a small amount of research that shows that aripiprazole may be able to counter this side effect of increased prolactin.

Certain antipsychotics, such as ziprasidone and some older antipsychotics require periodic EKG monitoring.

It is important to remember that not everyone experiences any or all of these side effects. For a complete listing of side effects, please consult the medication pamphlet accompanying the medication.

Many of these antipsychotic medications are also available in monthly or biweekly long-acting injectable formulations, which can make it easier to have good symptom control without having to remember to take pills every day.

If you or your family member suffers from schizophrenia or another primary psychotic disorder, your psychiatrist or physician will work closely with you to find a medication and dose that is most suited for your body and condition.

What Else Can Help?

Early diagnosis and prompt treatment helps reduce debilitation from symptoms and enhances quality of life.

Regular follow up with a psychiatrist helps ensure that the medication dose and side effects are being monitored and are individually suited to an individual's condition.

Stopping medications is a significant risk factor for symptom worsening or relapse. Family members can play a key role in helping the affected individual manage their symptoms, and to follow up and adhere with psychiatric treatment.

Some mental health organizations have teams that go to the affected individual's home to ensure that the mental health and daily needs of the individual with schizophrenia are being fully addressed.

There is research that shows that individuals with schizophrenia are more likely to suffer from medical conditions, such as diabetes, hypertension, obesity or others that are more likely to go untreated. This is another area where family members can play a key role in ensuring regular primary care follow up to maintain optimal physical health and functioning.

Most people with schizophrenia are not violent. However, recent studies have shown that individuals suffering from active psychotic symptoms, especially paranoia, may be at a somewhat higher risk of hurting themselves and others due to their delusional beliefs and hallucinations. Early identification and treatment is all the more important in these cases.

People with schizophrenia may need social skills training, employment training and/or housing support.

Schizoaffective Disorder

Schizoaffective disorder involves psychotic symptoms along with a mood episode, such as a major depressive, manic or hypomanic episode for a significant portion of the illness. The psychotic symptoms include some key symptoms that can also be found in schizophrenia, such as delusions or hallucinations. Schizoaffective disorder may be characterized as depressed type or bipolar type, and significantly impairs functioning in occupational, social and/or family life.

In general, with proper treatment, individuals with schizoaffective disorder may be able to have a somewhat higher level of functioning over their lifetime, as compared to individuals with schizophrenia.

Treatment involves treatment of the psychotic symptoms in addition to treatment of the depressive or manic/hypomanic symptoms. Medication treatment is key. In addition, family education and support as well as supportive psychotherapy can be beneficial.

Without treatment, individuals with schizophrenia and schizoaffective disorder may be at risk for suicide, homelessness, medical problems, social isolation and other complications. Family members can be key sources of support and stability for these individuals, as these individuals often tend to stop treatment, mainly due to impaired reality testing and fluctuating/declining insight into their illness.

Delusional Disorder

This is a rare psychiatric condition. A person suffering from delusional disorder commonly does not exhibit other psychotic symptoms except delusions and may not appear to have a significant degree of impairment in overall life functioning.

What is a Delusion?

A delusion is a false, fixed belief. A delusion may be bizarre or non-bizarre. Delusions can be of varied kinds, such as delusion of grandiosity, infidelity, persecutory, somatic or other.

What is Usually Not a Delusion?

The term delusion is often used loosely. However, a delusion is a specific clinical entity.

A delusion is different from an overvalued idea which is a false belief that is not held with the same degree of rigidity as a delusion. An individual holding an overvalued idea is usually more open to reasoning, questioning or entertaining the notion that the belief may not be accurate or true.

A belief that is typically held by or falls within the normal range of an individual's culture is not a delusion, even though the belief may seem bizarre to people outside of that culture.

Treatment of Delusional Disorder:

This can be a difficult condition to treat. Antipsychotic medication and/or psychotherapy may be suitable interventions, depending on an individual's specific clinical condition, symptom severity and other factors.

Delirium: A Condition that May Look Like Schizophrenia, but, Is Not

Although delirium is a medical condition, I am talking about it in this book given it is a medical emergency and poses life-threatening risks, if not identified and treated in a timely manner.

Delirium is most commonly seen in ICU settings or among elderly people suffering from infections such as UTIs. An individual with delirium often experiences hallucinations, paranoia, confusion, fluctuations in attention and consciousness, and/or at times, agitation or even apathy.

What Can Help?

- Identification and treatment of the underlying cause is of utmost importance in any type of delirium.
- In certain situations, use of a very low dose antipsychotic may be deemed appropriate for short-term symptom control.
- Certain medications, especially benzodiazepines and anticholinergic medications (for example, 'benadryl') can increase risk of delirium. Simplification of an individual's medication regimen and reduction of polypharmacy may be done by an experienced physician, when appropriate.
- Reduction of excessive stimulation in the environment is recommended.

References:

American Academy of Child and Adolescent Psychiatry. Facts for Families Guide. Depression in Children and Teens. Retrieved April 8, 2018, from https://www.aacap.org/AACAP/Families_and_youth/ Facts_for_Families/FFF-Guide/The-Depressed-Child-004.aspx

American Academy of Family Physicians (AAFP). Retrieved April 8, 2018, from https://www.aafp.org/patient-care/clinical-recommendations/all/myocardial.html

The National Association of Anorexia Nervosa and Associated Disorders, Inc. (ANAD). Retrieved April 8, 2018, from http://www.anad.org/get-information/about-eating-disorders/eating-disorders-statistics/

Bhatia, R. 'Rule out these Causes of Inattention before diagnosing ADHD'. Current Psychiatry, 2016 October;15(10):32-C3.

Centers for Disease Control and Prevention. Attention-Deficit/Hyperactivity Disorder (ADHD). ADHD Home: Basic Information. Retrieved April 1, 2018, from https://www.cdc.gov/ncbddd/adhd/facts.html

Centers for Disease Control and Prevention. Healthy Aging. Retrieved April 8, 2018, from https://www.cdc.gov/aging/mentalhealth/depression.htm

Cornelius MD, Day NL. The Effects of Tobacco Use During and After Pregnancy on Exposed Children: Relevance of Findings for Alcohol Research. Alcohol Research & Health. Vol. 24, No. 4, 2000. Retrieved on April 8, 2018, from https://pubs.niaaa.nih.gov/publications/arh24-4/242-249.pdf

Desk Reference to the Diagnostic Criteria from DSM-5. American Psychiatric Association.

Kessler RC, Bromet EJ. The epidemiology of depression across cultures. *Annual review of public health*. 2013;34:119-138. doi:10.1146/annurev-publhealth-031912-114409.

Mattes, JA. Treating ADHD in Prison: Focus on Alpha-2 Agonists (Clonidine and Guanfacine). The Journal of the American Academy of Psychiatry and the Law. Volume 44, Number 2, 2016.

Medi-Cal. Department of Health Care Services. CA.GOV. Retrieved on April 8, 2018, from https://files.medi-cal.ca.gov/pubsdoco/dur/articles/dured_14_fdawa.asp

MGH Center for Women's Mental Health: Reproductive Psychiatry Resource and Information Center. Psychiatric Disorders during Pregnancy. Retrieved on April 15, 2018, from

https://womensmentalhealth.org/specialty-clinics/psychiatric-disorders-during-pregnancy/

National Institute of Mental Health. Health and Education. Mental Health Information. Depression. Retrieved on April 8, 2018, from https://www.nimh.nih.gov/health/topics/depression/index.shtml

National Institute of Mental Health. Health and Education. Publications. NIMH Answers Questions About Suicide. Retrieved on April 8, 2018, from https://www.nimh.nih.gov/health/publications/nimh-answers-questions-about-suicide/index.shtml

National Institute of Mental Health. Health and Education. Mental Health Information. Brain Stimulation Therapies. Retrieved on April 8, 2018, from https://www.nimh.nih.gov/health/topics/brain-stimulation-therapies/brain-stimulation-therapies.shtml

World Health Organization (April 2017). Mental Disorders Fact Sheet. Retrieved April 1, 2018, from http://www.who.int/mediacentre/factsheets/fs396/en/